Successful Stress Management.

A Nutritional Guide - How to Achieve Stress Relief Through Your Diet.

By Laura Hails

Contents

Introduction

The food we eat creates the person that we become, eat healthy, nutritious food and you will look radiant, have more energy, sleep more soundly, become more active, lose excess weight and ultimately, achieve more. There is no doubt that introducing small changes into your daily routine coupled with daily exercise and the right diet can have dramatic results in our wellbeing.

Studies have shown that people who change their diets to a more healthy, nutritious one whilst dumping the junk and getting more exercise can significantly reduce levels of stress.

Too much stress over too long a period not only depletes your body of nutrients, leaving it exhausted, it also alters your body's biochemistry, making you more likely to crave and overeat junk food and store weight.

The De-Stress Diet uses healthy, nutritious food, so you have fewer cravings and produce a steady stream of feel-good chemicals naturally. As a bonus, you can lose weight and see your mood, skin and muscle tone improve.

This book will explain what a nutritious diet should look like, tips on how to introduce a healthy diet into your life and the foods that you should be consuming more of to help you feel calmer and more able to deal with the stresses in your life.

If you find this book helpful, please look out for my - "Successful Stress Management, Recipe Book" with loads of easy to follow, delicious recipes created specifically to help you combat stress.

Chapter One
Stress

This book is primarily about making healthy changes to your diet and incorporating more of the specific foods that we know help to relieve stress. What a healthy diet looks like and how to change yours for the better is discuss in later chapters, however before looking at your diet I think it is worth also looking at the possible causes of stress and ways of helping you manage it.

The effects of stress on your body

Stress is the body's reaction to any adverse

changes in our lifestyle whether physical, mental or emotional. Many events that happen to us put stress on our body.

Stress is a normal part of life, the human body is designed to experience stress and react to it. Stress can be positive, keeping you alert and ready to avoid danger but it becomes negative when a person faces continuous challenges without relief or relaxation between them. As a result, a person may become overworked, and stress-related tension builds.

Stress that continues without relief can lead to a condition called distress, a negative stress reaction. Distress can lead to physical problems including headaches, upset stomach, elevated blood pressure, chest pain and trouble sleeping. Research suggests that stress can also bring on or worsen certain symptoms and diseases.

Stress also becomes harmful when people turn to alcohol, tobacco, or drugs to try to relieve their stress. Unfortunately, instead of relieving the stress and returning the body to a relaxed state, these substances tend to keep the body in a stressed state and can cause more problems.

Stress can affect all aspects of your life, including your emotions, behaviour, thinking ability and physical health. No part of the body is immune, but because people handle stress differently, symptoms of stress can vary.

Emotional symptoms of stress include:

Easily agitated, frustrated and moody.

Feeling overwhelmed.

Difficulty relaxing.

Feelings of ow self-esteem.

Avoiding others/ depressed.

Physical symptoms of stress include:

Low energy

Headaches

Insomnia

Upset stomach,
including diarrhoea, constipation, and nausea

Aches, pains, and tense muscles

Chest pain and rapid heartbeat

Frequent colds and infections

Cold or sweaty hands and feet

Excess sweating

Dry mouth and difficulty swallowing

What causes stress?

Big life changes often create stress. People usually see stress as related to difficult events such as dealing with illness, bereavement or redundancy but even happy events like having a baby or planning a wedding can cause stress.

Stress may be related to:

Work – such as, unemployment, a high workload or retirement.

Family – such as, divorce, relationship difficulties or caring for a relative.

Housing – such as, moving- house or problems with neighbours.

Personal issues – such as, coping with a serious illness, bereavement or financial problems

How to deal with stress

It's important to tackle the causes of stress in your life if you can. Avoiding problems rather than facing them can make things worse. It is also important to try to understand the difference between situations or events that you can change and those that you can't. If you can't change it look for ways to take your mind off it by focusing on things that bring you enjoyment.

When you can't prevent stress look for ways to manage it instead.

Other things that may help:

1 - Research shows that people who share their problems with friends or family members are less likely to suffer from stress or depression. A good support network of colleagues, friends and family can ease your troubles and help you see things in a different way.

2 – People who have interests and hobbies outside of their work environment tend to be less stressed at work. Take time to do things that you enjoy. Try to set aside one or two evenings a week for socialising, relaxing or pursuing a hobby. By consciously setting time aside you will be less likely to work overtime.

3 – Take a break or holiday. Even a short break away from whatever it is that is causing your stress can have significant effects on the level of stress you are experiencing. Taking a break allows you time to refocus.

4 – Research shows that people who take some form of regular exercise are less likely to suffer from stress and group exercise is even more beneficial. Try joining an exercise club that suits your level of fitness and is something you will enjoy.

5 – Try to take control of the "thing" that is causing you the stress. By taking control of the problem, you are instantly looking for a solution, which in itself will make you feel impowered rather than helpless. Ignoring it will only make it worse.

6 – Set yourself goals, no matter how small or seemingly insignificant. Setting goals will help you deal with the problem in stages rather than viewing it as impossible.

7 – Don't turn to alcohol, nicotine or caffeine as a crutch, not only will they not help solve the problem they may even create new ones.

8 – Look at ways to prioritise your time better. List out your daily tasks and aim to complete the worst one first, so that after that everything is possible. Leave the least important to last so that it doesn't matter if it isn't done.

9 – Gravitate towards those things that make you happy whether it is family, friends or activities, enjoy the peace and satisfaction they bring you.

10 – Make sure you get enough sleep. Sleep and stress are closely linked: being stressed leads to problems sleeping, and problems sleeping make you more prone to stress. Being sleep-deprived leads to many of the same hormonal changes and cravings as being stressed.

A recent study found that people who are sleep deprived will consume, on average, an extra 385 calories per day

Time-management

People who are stressed often complain of just not having enough time, learning how to manage your time more effectively will help you feel more relaxed and more in control and that in itself can have significant results when dealing with stress.

A balanced lifestyle brings clarity and focus.

1 – <u>Set goals</u> in your personal life as well as your working one and take positive steps each day towards them – whether they are short term ones or long term. Knowing your goals will help you plan better and if you know where you want to go you will be more likely to focus on getting there.

2 – <u>Make lists</u> so that you stay organised and focused instead of distracted. Lists should be made at the start of each day it will help you work out your priorities both at home and at work. Enjoy ticking them off as you complete them, this will give you a sense of achievement.

3 – <u>Take a lunch break</u>, even if it is just a walk around the block, taking a break refocuses the mind and makes you feel more energised and more productive. Looking forward to lunch makes the day more manageable.

4 – <u>Prioritise your to do list</u> into what must be done down to what doesn't. When you have prioritised it in terms of the most urgent first, try to get into the habit of tackling the task you least want to do first – that way anything else feels less stressful.

5 – <u>Prioritise what is important and what is not</u> - People with good time management ensure that they do everything that is classed as "important" first that way they lower the chances of tasks turning from important to urgent. It is the urgent tasks that cause the stress, by consciously reducing them you reduce the potential for stress.

6 – <u>keep on top of emails</u> - One study found that one in three office workers suffers from email stress. Making a decision the first time you open an email

is crucial for good time management.
Make a conscious effort to immediately
delete emails that are not needed.
Delegate those that someone else can
deal with, complete those that only take a
couple of minutes and set the rest aside.
Add the ones you have set aside to your
to do list and deal with them in the course
of your work load.

Breathing exercise for stress

This calming breathing technique for stress, anxiety and panic takes just a few minutes and can be done anywhere. You will get the most benefit if you do it regularly, as part of your daily routine. You can do it standing up, sitting in a chair that supports your back, or lying on a bed or yoga mat on the floor.

1 - Make yourself comfortable.

2 - If you are lying down, place your arms slightly away from your sides, palms down. Bend your knees so that your feet are flat on the floor hip width apart.

3 - If you are sitting, place your arms on the arms of the chair, feet flat on the floor hip width apart.

4 - Let your breath flow as deep down into your stomach as you can.

5 - Breathe in through your nose and out through your mouth.

6 - Breathe in and out gently and regularly - counting to four when you breathe in and again when you breathe out.

7 – Continue for 3 to 5 minutes.

Try to be more aware of your thoughts and feelings. Being aware of people or situations that have a negative impact on the way you are feeling means that you have more control over them and more control empowers you to deal with them more effectively.

Being in control of the negative and embracing the positive is an important step in the journey to greater happiness and inner peace.

Positively, embrace what you can change rather than dwelling on what you can't. When you look for positive solutions to the problem it ceases to be a problem.

With goals, comes plans and with plans come solutions. Solutions lead to inner peace and harmony.

Chapter Two
A Nutritional Diet

In the fight against any ailment your diet is key. Your diet effects every aspect of your life. And whilst eating well can't stop you from being made redundant or reduce your work load it can make you feel good, keep your head clear and focused, help you sleep better and ultimately be able to deal with stressful situations in a more productive way. With a clear mind and a healthy body, you are more likely to look for positive solutions then dwelling on things that you can't change.

Proteins

Protein is a powerful nutrient, it plays a major role in our body, building body tissue and making important hormones. Proteins are made up of a collection of 20 amino acids, these are divided into two - "essential" which are sourced from your food and "non-essential that are produced by your body.

Protein, will keep you fuller for longer, it will help you concentrate, reduce sugar cravings, give you energy and keep your hair, nails and bones strong. The protein in your body is constantly being broken down and replaced. The body does not store amino acids like it does carbohydrates and fats, so it needs a daily supply of amino acids to make new proteins. The protein in the food you eat is digested into amino acids that can be used to replace the protein in your body.

There are two different types of proteins in our diet, complete and incomplete. The difference between the two is determined by its amino acid composition.

Complete Proteins – These are proteins that supply all "essential amino acids" complete proteins come from foods such as eggs, milk, meat, fish and soy.

Complete proteins are great sauces of protein and should make up 75% of our daily protein intake, however you can combine incomplete proteins with complete proteins to ensure you are getting the complete range of "essential amino acids" in your diet.

Animal Derived Complete Proteins –

Meat, poultry, fish and shellfish all contain all the "essential" amino acids. Fish and shellfish are a particularly good source of complete protein because they are low fat and rich in essential minerals. Examples include shrimp, scallops, clams, tuna, salmon, mackerel, halibut, sardines and cod.

Vegetarian, Animal Derived Complete Proteins – Eggs and dairy products are also complete proteins, containing all essential amino acids. Examples are eggs, cheese and yoghurt. Quorn – although not derived from animals is a plant based complete protein but as it contains some dairy it cannot be classed as vegan.

Vegan, Plant Based Complete Proteins - Plant-based foods that are complete protein choices, include soy products, quinoa and buckwheat – which are a protein-rich wholegrain. Soybeans form the basis of many processed soy foods, all of which are complete protein sources such as soy milk, tempeh, tofu, miso and

, edamame which are fresh green soybeans.

Incomplete Proteins – These are proteins that do not contain all essential amino acids, or don't have sufficient quantities of them to meet the body's needs and should be combined with other proteins. Examples of incomplete proteins are nuts and seeds, pulses, grains such as rice and vegetables.

These proteins shouldn't be ignored as they contribute towards a healthy, balanced diet. Proteins that in combination with each other provide the complete range of essential amino acids are called complementary proteins. Complimentary proteins don't have to be combined at the same meal, but they should be combined within the same day as the body does not store the protein it consumes.

Examples of complementary proteins are – rice and beans, spinach and almonds, hummus and whole grain pittas.

Carbohydrates –

Dietary carbohydrates are split into three categories:

Sugars – these are short chain carbohydrates that are found in foods, examples of sugar carbohydrates are glucose,

Starches – these are long chains of glucose molecules, which eventually get broken down into glucose in the digestive system these are found in potatoes, corn and oats, peas and rice.

Fibre – Humans cannot digest fibre, but the bacteria in the digestive system can make use of some of them, fibre is essential for a healthy digestive system. Fibre is found in vegetables, fruit, salad, pulses and whole grains.

The most important thing to know about carbohydrates is that you need them to give you energy, by eating the right foods you naturally become more energetic, you do more, and you burn off more calories. A balanced diet helps with weight control, sleeping patterns and memory and concentration levels. The key is to eat the right carbs and ditch the wrong ones

Carbohydrates in their natural form are good for you and should be part of a healthy, balanced diet. Whilst cutting down on simple carbohydrates such as biscuits, cakes and pastries will increase your wellbeing and help you maintain a healthy diet you shouldn't be tempted to cut complex carbohydrates from your diet.

Carbohydrates are not essential as the body can function without them, however, complex carbohydrates are an important part of a healthy diet because of their high nutritional value. Cut back on simple carbohydrates and increase the complex ones.

The More Complex the better

Complex Carbs are starch and fibre and have more nutrients then Simple Carbs. They have a higher fibre content and therefore, digest more slowly making you feel fuller for longer.

Complex carbohydrates are more filling and therefore will help you control your weight, they also help keep your blood sugars level, which stops cravings.

Complex Carbohydrates you should be eating – fruit, vegetables, nuts, pulses and whole grains, whole wheat bread and cereal,corn, oats, peas and brown or wild rice.

1 - whole grains – these are good sources of fibre, as well as potassium, magnesium and selenium. Choose - quinoa, buckwheat, and whole – wheat pasta and noodles

2 - Fruit – such as apples, berries and bananas.

3 - Vegetables – all vegetables, but in particular, leafy greens such as spinach, kale and cabbage.

4 - Beans – beans, peas and lentils.

Fats –

Good fats – Oil rich, nutritious foods like <u>nuts, seeds and avocados</u> are rich in omega 3 and 6 fatty acids which protect against heart disease, aid weight loss, lower cholesterol and promote healthy hair, nails and skin. Another way to get essential fat is to use cold pressed oils such as rapeseed, extra virgin olive oil, walnut and sesame oil.

Chapter Three
Eat the Rainbow

Antioxidants

Antioxidants come up frequently in discussions about good health and preventing diseases. These powerful substances, which mostly come from the fresh fruits and vegetables we eat, prohibit (and in some cases even prevent), the oxidation of other molecules in the body. The benefits of antioxidants are very important to good health, because if free radicals are left unchallenged, they can cause a wide range of illnesses and chronic diseases.

Antioxidants and Free Radicals

The human body naturally produces free radicals and the antioxidants to counteract their damaging effects. However, in most cases, free radicals far outnumber the naturally occurring antioxidants. In order to maintain the balance, and maximise the benefits of antioxidants a continual supply of external sources of antioxidants are necessary. Antioxidants benefit the body by neutralising and removing the free radicals from the bloodstream.

Different Antioxidants Benefit Different Parts of the Body

There are a wide range of antioxidants found in nature, and because they are so varied, different antioxidants provide benefits to different parts of the body. For example, beta-carotene (and other carotenoids) is very beneficial for healthy eyes, lycopene is beneficial for helping maintain

©prostate health; flavonoids are especially beneficial in maintaining a healthy heart; and proanthocyanins are beneficial for urinary tract health.

Antioxidants and Skin Health Benefits

When skin is exposed to high levels of ultraviolet light, photo-oxidative damage is induced by the formation of different types of reactive species of oxygen, including singlet oxygen, superoxide radicals, and peroxide radicals. These forms of reactive oxygen damage cellular lipids, proteins, and DNA, and they are considered to be the primary contributors to erythema (sunburn), premature aging of the skin, photo dermatoses, and skin cancers.

Antioxidants and Immune System Support

Singlet oxygen can compromise the immune

system, because it has the ability to catalyze production of free radicals. Astaxanthin and Spirulina have been shown to enhance both the non-specific and specific immune system, and to protect cell membranes and cellular DNA from mutation. Astaxanthin is the single most powerful quencher of singlet oxygen,and is up to ten times stronger than other carotenoids (including beta-carotene), and up to 500 times stronger than alpha tocopherol (Vitamin E), while Spirulina has a variety of antioxidants and other substances that are beneficial in boosting immunity.

Additional Ways Antioxidants Help Benefit our Health

Increasing one's antioxidant intake is essential for optimum health, especially in today's polluted world. Because the body just can't keep up with antioxidant production, a good amount of these vitamins, minerals, phytochemicals, and enzymes must come from our daily diet. Boosting your antioxidant intake can help provide added protection for the body against heart problems, eye problems, memory problems, mood disorders and immune system problems.

Top Antioxidant – rich Fruit and Vegetables.

Blackberries, blueberries, broccoli, Brussel sprouts, Curly kale, garlic, plums, prunes, raisins, raspberries, red peppers, spinach and strawberries.

Plant Nutrients -

The more variety and colour you eat the more nutrients you will consume and the more benefit you will get from your diet.

According to a recent National Diet and Nutrition Survey many of our diets - adults and children –

are lacking in vitamin A and D, selenium and zinc and many women are lacking calcium and iron.

Fruit and vegetables are considered so good for us that nutritionists suggest that the recommended government 5 a day should be our bare minimum. But the truth is that most people aren't even eating 5 a day. Fruit and vegetables provide a huge variety of vitamins, minerals and fibre and if you are missing out on eating them you will leave a big gap in the nutrients you consume.

The best way to get the most from your food is variety. Many people get stuck in a rut, eating the same food day in and day out with little or no variety. In order to stay healthy, the body needs over 40 different vitamins and minerals a day so sticking to the same foods will hugely reduce your intake.

Introducing new and different foods to your weekly shop will not only keep your food exciting but your body will reap the rewards.

Whilst some foods have significant health benefits it is important to remember that no one individual food can treat, prevent or cure health problems, the key is to eat all foods as part of a balanced diet.

Include fruit and vegetables from the five colour groups, red, orange, yellow, green and purple. Different coloured fruit and vegetables contain different nutrients, combining them is the best way to ensure you get all you need.

Many of the naturally occurring chemicals responsible for giving fruit and veg their bright colours actually help keep us healthy and free from disease. Fruit and vegetables contain hundreds of colourful phytochemicals that act as antioxidants.

Antioxidant-rich fruit and vegetables can help to protect against heart disease, cancer, and premature aging.

Red–

Many red foods contain high levels of vitamin C. They contain high levels of anthocyanins which are linked to being effective in fighting cancer, bacterial infections and neurological diseases.

Red fruit and vegetables to include in your diet are raspberries, cranberries, strawberries, cherries, pomegranate, apples, rhubarb, red peppers, tomatoes and watermelon.

Orange

Orange fruit and vegetables are high in carotenoids, crucial for maintaining a good immune system and supporting cell repair and healthy vision.

Orange fruit and vegetables to include in your diet are Carrots, oranges, squashes, sweet potatoes, mangoes, peaches, nectarines, pumpkins, swede and peppers.

Yellow

Yellow fruit and vegetables contain large amounts of bioflavonoids, which fight infection and reduce inflammation.

Yellow fruit and vegetables to introduce into your diet – corn, pineapple, peppers and squashes.

Green

Green fruit and vegetables contain nutrients including lutein, lycopene, folic acid, zeaxanthin and glycosylates all of which are associated with helping to prevent cancer.

Green fruit and vegetables to include in your diet

- asparagus, avocado, rocket, spinach, lettuce, watercress, cucumber, broccoli, Brussels sprouts, leafy cabbage, spring greens, beans, peas, sugar snap peas, mange tout, cress, courgette, peppers, spring onions, leeks, apples, grapes and kiwi fruit.

Purple/blue

Purple and blue fruit and vegetables are high in antioxidants which promote healthy blood and are believed to have antiaging properties.

Purple and blue fruit and vegetables to include in your diet are blackberries, blueberries, grapes, blackcurrants, plums, red cabbage, prunes, red onions, olives, purple sprouting broccoli, beetroot and aubergine.

Chapter Four
A Balanced Plate

Eat more than just the rainbow - As well as a variety of fruit, salad and vegetables we should also be eating beans, fish, nuts and seeds and good oils.

Beans –

Also known as pulses or legumes, pulses are packed with complete protein and contain almost no fat and are a good source of complex carbohydrates which are essential for good health.

Studies have linked that a higher consumption of

beans results in a lower risk of heart disease and developing type 2 diabetes. It is now believed that a good intake of beans probably reduces the risk of stomach and prostate cancer.

Beans are low in fat and saturates and are packed with insoluble and soluble fibre, protein and a variety of minerals. Insoluble fibre helps keep our digestive system healthy whilst soluble fibre helps to control blood sugar levels and lowers cholesterol which means a lower risk of heart disease.

Beans provide potassium a nutrient that helps maintain fluid balance and helps to lower blood pressure. They also contain magnesium and phosphorus which strengthen bones. Many beans contain copper which gives us healthy skin and hair as well as a healthy immune system heart. Most beans provide manganese which is important for brain function and the metabolism of carbs and fat.

Beans are high in protein as well as good source of iron which makes them perfect for vegetarians and vegans. Because they contain both protein and fibre they keep us feeling fuller for longer. They help to slow down the absorption of sugar into the blood which means sugar levels stay even, this is not only good news for people trying to lose weight as it controls the appetite but also good news for people with type 2 diabetes who need to prevent dramatic rises in blood sugar.

Choose from - Aduki beans, black eyed beans, borlotti beans, chickpeas, fava beans, haricot beans, kidney beans, lentils, mung beans, soybeans and split peas.

Nuts –

There are many health benefits to eating nuts they help lower your cholesterol, lower blood pressure and help you lose weight. The high fat content in nuts make them good for your heart because they are rich in polyunsaturated and monounsaturated fats which lower cholesterol.

Almonds – contain the most fibre, calcium and vitamin B2 which are good for healthy bones, skin, eyesight, red blood cells, nervous system and digestive system.

Brazil Nuts – have a very high selenium content, which is an antioxidant that is essential for a healthy immune system and protects against disease causing free radical damage.

Cashew Nuts – contain the most iron and make them a brilliant choice for vegetarians. Eat with vitamin C rich foods or a glass of orange juice to help the body absorb the iron more easily.

Peanuts – contain the least amount of calories and fat but the most amount of protein and B vitamins. Studies have also shown that people who ate a handful of peanuts twice a week significantly reduced their risk of bowel cancer.

Pistachios – has one of the lowest calories and fat content of other nuts and are the only nut to contain an antioxidant called lutein. Lutein is found in green vegetables and is good for healthy eyes.

Walnuts – are a great source of omega 3, walnuts contain alpha- linolenic acid which the body uses to make omega 3 fats that are found in oily fish such as salmon and mackerel.

Seeds –

Seeds are high in fats that are good for the heart as well as containing beneficial vitamins such as A, B, C, and E and nutrients such as iron, potassium, magnesium, phosphorus, copper, zinc and manganese. Just 30g of pumpkin seeds contain six times more iron then a small roasted chicken and 15% more than a small grilled rump steak, which makes them brilliant for vegetarians and vegans.

Sunflower seeds, flax seeds, alfalfa seeds, pumpkin seeds and sesame seeds are particularly beneficial. Seeds are so nutrient-dense that you don't have to eat a lot of them. Use them in cooking as garnishes or to flavour stews and casseroles, sprinkle them on soup, salads and roasted vegetables. Add them to cereals or smoothies or eat them as a snack.

Grains –

Grains are rich in nutrients and are basic energy foods. Almost all whole, unrefined grains can be beneficial to your health, generally the darker the colour the healthier it is.

Barley – pot barley is the wholegrain version. Barley is good for digestion. It is low in gluten.

Brown Rice – is beneficial for the nervous system and digestive system. It is the least allergenic of all grains. Basmati is perfect for people are overweight.

Buckwheat – is gluten free and rich in healthy minerals. A perfect choice for people who are sensitive to wheat. It is a good source of protein.

Millet – is high in iron, magnesium, potassium, the B vitamins and vitamin E. Millet helps to support the digestive system, improves nutrient uptake and is a great energy booster.

Quinoa – comes from South America. It contains all the essential amino acids and is therefore, a complete protein but is easier to digest than meat protein and contains less fat.

Oats – contain more good fats then other grains. They are also a good source of vitamin B Complex which is good for the nervous system and for strengthening bones.

Spelt – like buckwheat is packed with minerals and protein. It is a good alternative for people who are sensitive to wheat, it helps stimulate the immune system and provides a good source of constant energy.

Fish –

Eating more fish is an important part of a healthy diet. Fish is a good source of protein. White fish and shellfish are low in fat and therefore low in calories. Studies have linked good intakes of fish with a reduced risk of heart disease, depression, dementia and Alzheimer's disease.

There is evidence that eating more fish may even reduce the risk of certain cancers.

<u>White Fish</u> – have a significant amount of B vitamins. White fish also contains iodine and selenium, nutrients that are essential for a healthy immune system.

Plaice – is particularly high in biotin which is needed for healthy hair and nails.

Sea Bream – is good for boosting vitamin B6 which is needed for making red blood cells.

Halibut – is one of the best sources of vitamin B3 which is essential for a healthy nervous system and releases energy from food.

Lemon sole and haddock – are good sources of iodine.

<u>**Oil Rich Fish**</u> – are packed with omega 3 fats which help prevent heart disease, heart attacks and strokes. Omega 3 fats are important for brain cell development particularly before babies are born and in the first few years of childhood.

Oily fish are also rich in vitamin D a nutrient that helps the body absorb calcium which keeps bones strong.

Sardines – not only contain calcium but also high levels of vitamin D.

Tuna (fresh not tinned) – contains high levels of selenium and iron which is an important nutrient for healthy blood.

Salmon – contains good amounts of omega 3 fats as well as being a particularly good source of vitamin E and vitamin B6.

Mackerel – contains one of the richest sources of omega 3 fats as well as iodine and vitamin D.

Shellfish – provide zinc which is essential for normal growth, enzyme function, wound healing, fertility and a healthy immune system.

Scallops – are particularly nutritious, they contain more selenium than either white fish or oily fish and tend to have more iron.

Muscles – are also a good source of iron.

Crab – is a good source of copper which is an important mineral for healthy hear and skin as well as a healthy immune and nervous system.

Prawns – have a higher cholesterol content then other fish but the cholesterol levels in prawns has little effect on blood cholesterol in the body and it is far more important to cut down on saturated fats.

Good Oils –

There are many different types of oils on the market, choosing the right one will bring nutritional value to your cooking.

On the whole oils contain less saturated fat then animal fats such as butter and lard. And more polyunsaturated and monounsaturated fats which can lower your cholesterol.

Cooking oils which are liquid when kept at room temperature are mostly derived from plants, nuts and seeds. They all have a similar amount of calories, which is approx. 100kcal per 1 tbsp. but they differ in the type of fat they contain and their smoke point, which is the temperature at which they start to break down. When the smoke point is reached, the quality, flavour and nutritional benefits are affected. It is important to understand what oils are best for what type of use.

Ground Nut Oil – is made from peanuts and is wonderful for your heart. It is packed with plant sterols that can lower your risk of heart disease. Ground nut oil – as its name would suggest – has a slightly nutty but mild flavour and is very versatile. It has a high smoke point which makes it a good oil to use for grilling or frying.

Olive Oil – is rich in monounsaturated fats which boost good cholesterol and have a beneficial effect on your heart. Olive oil can be heated to higher temperatures which makes it perfect for grilling, baking, roasting or stirring through pastas.

Light Olive Oil – means that the oil is lighter

in colour and flavour and it has a higher smoke point making it good for grilling and frying. The term "light" does not mean that it contains fewer calories or fat content.

Extra Virgin Olive Oil – is richer in antioxidants. It has a lower smoke point which means that it loses much of its nutritional benefits when heated. Use it for dressing and sauces that don't need to be cooked.

Rapeseed Oil – is a good all-rounder. Low in saturated fats and high in heart friendly monounsaturated fats rapeseed oil also contains omega 3 and vitamin E. This oil is great in salad dressings but also, because it has a high smoke point it is also perfect for frying, roasting and baking.

Sunflower Oil – is low in saturated fats, rich in polyunsaturated fat – omega 6, and vitamin E. It is a good all-purpose oil, its mild flavour makes it good for using in salads and dressings and its high smoke point means it is also good for frying, roasting and grilling.

Toasted Sesame Oil – is most associated with oriental dishes because of its rich, nutty flavour. It is a good sauce of oleic acid which is good for the heart. Its low smoke point means it is not good for cooking – unless you combine it with another oil, such as Olive or Sunflower oil. It is best used for its flavour in salad dressings or dips.

Chapter Five

Rules for Healthy Living.

Cook from scratch

Take responsibility for what you are eating by knowing exactly what is in your food. Cooking from scratch doesn't have to be complicated or time consuming. look for quick, simple recipes, the fewer the ingredients the quicker the dish, and use good quality ingredients to maximise nutrition. Plan ahead and know what you are going to cook and adapt your menu to the time you have. The recipes in this plan will help you do just that.

Read the labels

Food labels are a reliable, accurate source of valuable nutritional information. Use the labels on the foods you buy to ensure that you are consuming what you think you are consuming. Ingredients are listed in descending order by weight and include any colour, additives, preservatives and, nutrients, fats or sugar that have been added to the product.

Whatever appears first on the list is the largest ingredient. Foods with high levels of sugar, salt or saturated fats at the top of the list should be avoided.

Know your Sugar

Sugar comes in many forms with many different names, but it is all the same and has the same effect on the body. Products with sugar listed at the top of its ingredients list is more than likely high in sugar. The following are all sugars – brown sugar, cane juice lactose, maltose, raw cane sugar, raw sugar, sucrose sugar, invert sugar, glucose, fructose, dextrose, corn syrup, corn sweetener.

Consider naturally sweet alternatives such as raw honey or maple syrup or add fruit such as apples, apricots and berries. Carrot or apple juice makes a great base for vegetable juices as they add sweetness.

Know Your Fats

Good fats or "essential fatty acids" as they are known come from nuts and seeds, fish and avocados, they are important for a healthy, balanced diet. These can also be added to your cooking by using them as oils such as sunflower and pumpkin seed oil, macadamia, coconut, walnut, hazelnut and olive oils are all beneficial fats that support nerve function, mental alertness, concentration and memory.

Bad fats or saturated / trans fats are known to raise levels of cholesterol and increase the risk of heart disease. These are found mainly in animal produce and dairy products they are in butter, lard, margarine, cooking fats, chocolate, biscuits, cakes, savory snacks and processed foods.

Read the label and avoid anything that says it contains "hydrogenated" or "partially hydrogenated oils"

Add colour

The more colour in your diet the more goodness you will consume. Each colour of fruit and vegetables contain different and important antioxidants. Antioxidants are part of a well-balanced, healthy diet, they will keep you well throughout the winter months by helping your immune system to kill harmful bacteria and infections and they will keep your skin and hair looking good and give you vitality. Vitamins A, C and E are all found in fresh fruit and vegetables and are all antioxidants.

Be prepared

Always make a meal plan and a shopping list before shopping. Consider the week ahead in advance. Think about foods that you love and how you can introduce more variety to them. Don't be afraid to find recipes and tweak them to suit your own tastes you may discover something wonderful.

Consider days that you might be home late or have more work to do than normal and make those evening meals simple and quick or even prepare them at the weekend, or when you have more time, and freeze them so that they are at hand when you need a quick meal. Making your own microwave meals doesn't need to be either complicated or time consuming – it just needs planning. Consider, omelets, stir fries or salads with fresh or tinned fish.

Stay Hydrated

Dehydration can, falsely, make you think that you are hungry. Your brain can confuse thirst with hunger. Before reaching for a biscuit or sweets make a conscious effort to have a glass of water and then decide whether you were hungry or thirsty. If you really are hungry consider what you are reaching for.

Healthy Snacking.

Snacking between meals is a good thing. As long as you make the right choices, healthy snacking keeps your blood sugars level and increases your energy. Snacking keeps your brain active meaning that you can concentrate and remain focused throughout the day and on into the evening.

If you enjoy your snacks, aim for fruit, plain or unsweetened Greek-style yogurt, celery sticks, carrots or nuts and seeds.

Not Just 5 a Day

We all know that 5 portions of fruit and vegetables a day is the recommended amount. Given the nutritional value in fruit and vegetables and the health benefits of them 5 portions should be your absolute minimum and whilst meal planning you should be looking at ways of increasing your consumption wherever you can.

Try adding fruit to your breakfast cereal or drinking a smoothie instead of a cup of tea for breakfast, be more adventurous with your salads, replace your lunchtime sandwich and crisps with a salad and add vegetables to your pasta sauces, stews and soups and before you know it you will have increased your intake of fruit and veg without even noticing.

Flavour Your Food with Herbs and Spices.

Spices have been found to inhibit the formation of prostaglandins – the hormones that trigger inflammatory reactions. Reduce your use of salt and increase your use of herbs and mild spices to flavour your food instead. Use - cloves, cinnamon, turmeric, rosemary, ginger, sage, and thyme all of which are known for their anti-inflammatory properties.

Scientists in India have found that curcumin, the primary active ingredient of turmeric, has anti – depressant qualities that were found to be at least as effective as certain medications in the treatment of depression – but without the negative side effects.

Refined V Unrefined

Always choose unrefined ingredients over refined ones.

Unrefined foods contain more natural nutrients because they have not been stripped of their vitamins and minerals in the refining process.

Fibre

People who eat a lot of refined foods and skip the fruit and vegetables are missing out on fibre. A lack of fibre in the diet leads to digestive problems and blood sugar imbalances. Fibre is the indigestible portion of grains, vegetables and fruit it is used by the body to improve intestinal function, helps to grow healthy bacteria in the gut and helps prevent disease by removing waste products and toxins from the body. Drop the white bread, pasta and rice and increase fruit, vegetables and whole grains wherever possible.

Eat at least 25 grams of fibre every day. A fibre-rich diet helps reduce inflammation by supplying the body with anti-inflammatory phytonutrients found in fruits, vegetables, and other whole foods. The best sources of fibre are whole grains, such as barley and oatmeal; vegetables such as peas, Brussel sprouts, parsnips and spinach, and fruit such as apples, bananas, oranges, strawberries and raspberries.

Chapter Six
Blood Sugar Balance

One of the reasons the food you eat determines your mood is because having too much or too little sugar in your blood can be stressful for your brain.

From an evolutionary point of view, both are perceived as a threat to your survival. Too much sugar happens when you eat a high-carb meal or snack (fruit juice, a bowl of cereal, a doughnut, a "health" bar), which is broken down rapidly into glucose and increases the amount of sugar in your blood.

A steep rise in blood sugar makes you feel

mentally good (sugar high) but persistent high blood sugar can be dangerous and lead to complications like hyperglycaemia, which is why the body has a fast and effective way of bringing blood sugar back down, using insulin.

Insulin takes sugar out of your blood into your liver and muscles for temporary safe storage. The resulting sudden dip in blood sugar is what makes you feel lethargic and foggy-brained (afternoon slump), which is when your adrenals have to kick in and secrete fight-or-flight hormones that quicken your breathing, make your heart race, and rev up your anxiety.

This is usually when you reach for one or all of the following: chocolate, more coffee, a salty carb snack, alcohol, drugs, cigarettes. It's got very little to do with self-control. When you're up against low blood sugar and an exhausted brain, the odds are against you.

This roller-coaster adrenal trip is exhausting for

your brain and alters your hormones. For most people, the roller coaster of extremes continues throughout their life until they eventually tire out their pancreas (diabetes), their adrenals (adrenal fatigue), and their brain (Alzheimer's disease).

The good news is you can prevent these diseases and take better care of your brain by making healthier choices.

Stress can be caused by several internal and external factors, but there's a natural way to manage it that many people don't realise.

The nutritional strategy known as blood sugar balance is a straightforward technique that involves eating fats and proteins at every meal and snack and avoiding sugar and stimulants as much as possible.

It is that simple. And it's also the only effective way to sustainably lose weight.

You should aim to eat protein at each meal, such as, fish, eggs, nuts, whole-fat dairy or beans and lentils. With your protein eat a variety of low-starch vegetables. Eating a mix of cooked and raw vegetables ensures variety as well as getting the best from your diet in terms of nutrients.

Healthy fats Omega oils or polyunsaturated fats should make up the main part of your fat intake, especially omega-3 oils from oily fish and eggs as well as monounsaturated fatty acids which you can get from avocados, olives and olive oil, nuts and seeds. Have two to three pieces of fresh fruit a day.

Avoid drinks that are high in sugar or caffeine and try instead, to for water, green tea and herbal teas.

Meal ideas to help with stress relief

Breakfast

- One or two poached, boiled or scrambled eggs with smoked salmon, avocado and sourdough rye bread.

- Baked beans with wilted spinach.

- Burcher Muesli - rolled oats, nuts and seeds soaked in water or yoghurt, mixed with apple and berries.

Lunch

- Vegetable and bean soup.

- Grilled fish with a green salad.

- Smashed avocado on wholegrain toast with a mixed salad.

- Roast mixed vegetables.

- Mixed bean salad.

Dinner

- Green Leaves and Cashew nut Stir-fry.

- Lentil dahl with steamed veggies.

- Grilled fish with a mixed green salad.

- Mixed bean stew

- Baked sweet potatoes with cottage cheese and mixed salad.

Snacks

- A piece of fruit.

- Handful of nuts and seeds.

- Hearty Smoothie

- Humous or natural yoghurt and crudities

Chapter Seven

Foods that De-Stress

Whilst a healthy, balanced diet is the key to fighting all ailments, there are specific foods that are known to combat specific conditions. Below is a list of foods that will specifically help de-stress you. Aim to include more of them in your daily menu.

Recommended foods

Almonds

Almonds are packed full of vitamins, vitamin E to bolster the immune system plus B vitamins which are known to make the body more able to deal with bouts of stress and depression.

Avocados

These wonderful fruits are rich in glutathione, a substance that blocks intestinal absorption of certain fats that cause oxidative damage. They also contain lutein, beta-carotene, vitamin E and more folate than any other fruit as well as vitamin B. Avocados are high in fat so whilst their health benefits are fantastic they are also high in calories.

Asparagus

Asparagus is high in folate, which is essential for keeping you calm.

Beetroot

Beetroot appears to be a powerful dietary source

of health promoting agents. Because of the powerful antioxidants in beetroot it has increased in popularity and is used more and more as a nutritional approach to help manage heart disease and cancer. Research shows that beetroot can reduce blood pressure, reduce inflammation and reduce levels of stress.

Berries

Berries contain some of the highest levels of antioxidants and have been linked to many positive health benefits. All berries are rich in vitamin C which has been shown to help combat stress. Studies have shown that after taking vitamin C people showed fewer signs of stress i.e. raised blood pressure, after a stressful event than those who had not taken the vitamin.

Brazil Nuts

Brazil nuts contain exceptionally high levels of selenium, which is a mineral that plays a key role in your metabolism. Research has also shown that selenium can reduce feelings of depression and help to boost your overall mood. Adequately incorporating selenium into your diet will not only put you in a better mood,but will help you feel more able to deal with stressful situations.

Broccoli

Broccoli is packed with vitamins, including stress-fighting B vitamins and folic acid. These nutrients relieve stress, anxiety, and depression. To preserve these vitamins and get the most out of what broccoli has to offer, enjoy it raw in salads and stir fries.

Brussel Sprouts

Brussels sprouts have omega-3 fatty acids, which research suggests may boost brain health, lower blood pressure, prevent heart disease, and help treat depression. Omega-3, is also found in oily fish, nuts, seeds.

Cannellini Beans

Also known as white beans cannellini beans can help with stress. Cannellini beans are rich in phosphatidylserine, a chemical that helps with cellular function in the brain. They are high in resistant starch, which can help to regulate blood sugar levels which helps reduce the symptoms of stress.

Carrots

Chronic stress can weaken our ability to fight disease. By upping our intake of antioxidant-rich fruits and vegetables, we can boost our immune system. Acorn squash and carrots, for example, are great sources of beta-carotene a stress busting antioxidant.

Cashews

Cashews, like all nuts are a good combination of protein and fat and are therefore very healthy, though like avocados they are high in calories so consider how much you are consuming. Cashews are a good source of zinc; low levels of zinc are linked to anxiety and depression which is also linked to stress. Our bodies don't store zinc it is important to get it from our diet.

Chamomile Tea

Chamomile tea is one of the most highly recommended drinks to have before bed as it aids a restful sleep. Studies have shown that people who took chamomile in a supplement form for 8 weeks showed significant signs of reduced stress and anxiety.

Dark Chocolate

Dark chocolate contains healthy antioxidants which help maintain a healthy heart. There is an undeniable link between chocolate and mood. Research has shown that in moderation, chocolate does make you feel better. Dark chocolate is known to lower blood pressure which has a calming effect.

Fish

Omega-3 fatty acids are powerful nutrients that increase serotonin, and you can find them in abundance in fatty fish like salmon and tuna. They actually work to prevent stress hormone surges and combat heart disease, depression and premenstrual syndrome (PMS). There's even a study that says omega-3s can lower anxiety associated with pregnancy.

Garlic

Garlic is packed with powerful antioxidants. These chemicals neutralise free radicals – particles that damage our cells, cause diseases and encourage aging. Studies show that antioxidants can help prevent some of the damage the free radicals cause over time. Garlic contains allicin, which research suggests may help the body fight off heart disease and cancer.

Because prolonged bouts of stress weaken the immune system, garlic can help strengthen it again.

Green Tea

Green tea contains an amino acid called L-theanine which is known to relieve stress and promote relaxation. It is also known to protect against some forms of cancer and enhance mental performance. Drink green tea instead of coffee which is known as a stimulant that interferes with blood sugar and spikes your stress hormones.

Kale

Dark leafy greens like kale are rich in folate, which helps your body produce mood-regulating neurotransmitters, including serotonin and dopamine. Folate prevents mental fatigue and forgetfulness by increasing blood flow to the brain. Most, antidepressants focus on the production of serotonin. Give your happiness levels a boost by including spinach, kale, or other leafy greens into your diet.

Legumes

Beans are densely packed with essential nutrients and have recently been acknowledged as one of the richest foods in antioxidants.

Oatmeal

A complex carbohydrate, not only does it contain antioxidants, oatmeal causes your brain to produce serotonin, a feel-good chemical. Serotonin creates a calming feeling that helps you overcome stress. Studies have shown that people that eat oatmeal for breakfast stay sharper throughout the morning.

Onions

Onions contain a compound called quercetin which acts as a sedative which can help reduce pain, depression and anxiety which can lead to stress.

Oranges

Oranges, like all citrus fruits are packed with vitamin C. Vitamin C not only helps boost your immune system it is also known to lower blood pressure and reduce stress levels.

Oysters

Oysters are packed full of zinc, zinc plays a big part in keeping both the immune system and the nervous system healthy. Stress and anxiety deplete zinc.

Studies have shown that people who suffer from stress and anxiety have significantly lower plasma levels of zinc and higher levels of copper.

Pak Choi

Pak Choi is packed with vitamin-rich nutrients. It contains vitamin C, vitamin B6, folate and magnesium all known for their benefits in the bodies fight against stress.

Seaweed

Seaweed is a food that is known to make you happy, it is a great source of magnesium and tryptophan. Magnesium helps relax the muscles while tryptophan is an amino acid that helps produce serotonin which elevates your mood and reduces anxiety which leads to stress. If you would rather take it in supplement for it is called spirulina and can be found in health food shops.

Seeds

Seeds are full of health promoting and stress reducing benefits. Pumpkin seeds, like cashews, are rich in magnesium, which is important for a healthy nervous system. Sunflower seeds are full of tryptophan, an amino acid that aids in the production of serotonin and melatonin, both of which influence sleep and mood.

Spinach

Spinach is packed full of magnesium, which the body uses to maintain a healthy nervous system. People with a magnesium deficiency have a greater inability to cope with stress.

Walnuts

Walnuts contain alpha-linolenic acid, an essential omega-3 fatty acid and other polyphenols that have been shown to help prevent memory loss. Foods rich in omega-3 such as nuts, seeds and oily fish lowers inflammation and have been shown to reduce stress and anxiety.

Watercress

Research has shown that antioxidant – rich watercress can alleviate stress. Watercress is rich in B vitamins which help to relieve stress, treat anxiety and depression, aid in memory and relieve PMS. Some B vitamins also help cells burn fats and glucose for energy, whereas others help make serotonin the feel-good neurotransmitter created in our brain.

Chapter Eight

Foods to Avoid When Stresses

How Stress Can Lead to Weight Gain.

High-sugar, low-soluble-fibre carbohydrates such as junk foods and refined grains heighten the energy and mood highs and lows caused by stress hormones.

Too many carbohydrates from refined sugars, and too few from vegetables, fruit and nuts, can lead to inflammation and a heightened insulin response, which adds to the fat storage caused by raised stress hormones.

A stressed brain is in dire need of continual sugar as fuel, as well as salt and processed fats. These foods initially make us feel better, but then lead to a mood drop, as well as more cravings and long-term weight gain.

Dealing with Sugar Cravings

1 - Have a healthy protein snack just before 4pm, when blood-sugar levels and willpower are at their lowest. Protein keeps your blood sugars level.

2 – Increase the amount of healthy, quality proteins and fats in your diet such as fish, eggs, beans, nuts and seeds.

3 – Initially substitute sugar for Stevia or honey in tea and coffee but try to wean yourself off it over a few weeks.

4 - Have sweet-tasting foods that don't upset blood sugar, such as unsweetened coconut, natural vanilla essence and unsweetened apple puree.

Foods to Avoid –

1 – Caffeine

A stimulant – caffeine has long had a reputation for triggering the body's fight or flight response. Caffeine can lead to feelings of anxiety which leads to stress. If you drink a lot of caffeine try initially replacing one or two of your cups of coffee with a herbal or green tea. Over time try to reduce it further so that it becomes a treat rather than a crutch.

2 – Artificial and Refined Sugars

Research has shown that although sugar does not cause stress it does create changes in the body that can exacerbate anxiety symptoms and impairs the body's ability to effectively cope with stress. A sugar crash is similar to a caffeine crash, and can also cause mood changes, heart palpitations, difficulty concentrating and exhaustion all of which are linked to anxiety that often leads to stress.

3 – Gluten

Gluten is a protein found in wheat, barley and rye products. Gluten can be a trigger for anxiety symptoms. Research has shown that people with a gluten intolerance are at a higher risk of suffering from anxiety, depression and mood disorders all of which impairs the body's

ability to effectively cope with stress. Cutting gluten out of your diet could help deal with anxiety and therefore stress.

4 – Processed Food

Processed foods are known for containing numerous additives and preservatives. Refined flours and sugars feed the harmful bacteria and microbes in the gut. Research has now linked the gut to the brain. Gut health is a major contributor to mood disorders, anxiety and stress. Good bacteria in the gut means a healthy happy gut and a happy brain.

5 – Alcohol

Alcohol is said to induce the symptoms of anxiety. Alcohol is a toxin that leads to mental and physical alterations by negatively impacting the levels of serotonin in the brain. It also causes an increased heart rate, lowered blood sugar levels and dehydration.

6 – Fizzy Drinks

In addition to the artificial food colouring and additives found in some fizzy drinks, aspartame is one of the most common ingredients found in diet drinks. Aspartame blocks the production of serotonin in the brain and can be responsible for headaches, insomnia, mood swings and anxiety all of which either exacerbate stress or impair the body's ability to deal with it.

7 – Fried Foods

Fried foods are both difficult to digest and have very little nutritional value. Poor nutritional content couples with unhealthy cooking methods increases the symptoms of anxiety. Most fried foods are cooked in hydrogenated oil which, if eaten on a regular basis can lead to heart disease.

8 – Foods High in Salt

Salt is essential in maintaining good health and a balanced diet, but too much can trigger panic episodes and can lead to anxiety, panic and depression. Research shows that too much salt in our diet can have a negative effect on the body's neurological system, causing fatigue and damaging the immune system. A restful sleep is a major key to a healthy mind, mood and body. Too much salt in the diet also leads to weight gain, high blood pressure and water retention. Reduced calorie foods are often high in sugar and salt. Beware of reduced calorie diet foods which often contain abnormally high levels of salt and sugar.

9 - Spicy foods

Stressed is often linked to digestive problems. When the body is under stress the digestive system is not able to work properly and process food resulting in your metabolism slowing down and food stay in your stomach for longer. This, in turn, leads to acid reflux which are made worse when you eat spicy foods.

While the author has made every effort to ensure that the information contained in this book is as accurate and up to date as possible, it is advisory only and should not be used as an alternative to seeking specialist medical advice. The author cannot be held responsible for actions that may be taken by the reader as a result of reliance on the information contained in this book, which are taken entirely at the readers own risk.

www.ingramcontent.com/pod-product-compliance
Lightning Source LLC
Chambersburg PA
CBHW051757250726
48659CB00001B/465